The Diabetic Diary

The Diabetic Diary

2001

Larry D. Sutton

Writers Club Press
San Jose New York Lincoln Shanghai

The Diabetic Diary
2001

Writers Club Press
an imprint of iUniverse.com, Inc.

For information address:
iUniverse.com, Inc.
5220 S 16th, Ste. 200
Lincoln, NE 68512
www.iuniverse.com

ISBN: 0-595-17237-7

Printed in the United States of America

CONTENTS

LIST OF ABREVIATIONS

ALT ....Alanine aminotransferase
AST ....Aspartate aminotransferase
BMI..Body mass index
BUN ....Blood urea nitrogen
CK...Creatine Kinase
CRT ....Creatinine
dl ....deciliter
HDL-C..High density lipoprotein cholesterol
Hg ....Mercury
hr ....Hour
in ....inches
K ....Potassium
Kg ....Kilograms
lb. ....pounds
LDL-C ....Low density lipoprotein cholesterol
m..meters
mg ....Milligrams
min ....Minute
mm ....Millimeters
Trig ....Triglycerides
µg ....Micrograms

Introduction

Diabetes is a leading cause of illness and death affecting approximately 16 million Americans, and the number is growing as baby boomers mature to retirement.

The care of the diabetic patient has become extremely complex for both patient and physician. Current medical philosophy is to prevent or limit diabetic complications by vigilant surveillance and early intervention. It is therefore very important to ensure that no part of the diabetic care plan be omitted. Contrast this with a report that only 20% of physicians follow standardized guidelines for medical management!

The *Diary* was designed to efficiently aid the diabetic patient and his or her physician to achieve complete preventive and health maintenance standard of care. Preceding each section are explanations of current recommendations and instructions for using that particular section. The greatest weight was given to recommendations from the American Diabetic Association. It is not intended as a comprehensive treatise on diabetes. That is left to the literally hundreds of books on diabetes currently on the market.

By renewing the *Diary* yearly you will have a permanent annual record of your health information and management. Filling out the *Personal Information, Medical and Surgical History,* and *Current Medications* sections yearly allows any changes from the preceding year(s) to be made without the clutter that results from deleting and scribbling insertions onto your records. An illegible or poorly legible *Diary* may lead to suboptimal health delivery. Also, since today's medical information is accumulating at a frantic pace and changes in standard of care are likely, yearly renewal of this *Diary* allows for modifications in recommendations for diabetic care.

If the information in this Diary is kept current, it will serve as an invaluable aid in optimizing your health care delivery. It is therefore recommended that you bring this Diary with you to all physician encounters including emergency room visits.

This book is not intended to prescribe treatment. Because treatment must be individualized, you should consult with your physician for recommendations concerning your treatment requirements.

Thank you for choosing THE DIABETIC DIARY. It is an honor to be chosen to participate in your health care delivery.

PERSONAL INFORMATION

▶ Fill in the information as directed.

▶ Take this book with you for all physician and emergency room visits. The information in this section, and the Past Medical History and Medications sections provide important and sometimes critical information to health care providers concerning your medical management. The information as presented in this book is designed to be as efficient as possible for your physicians.

▶ Diabetes that was formerly referred to as Juvenile, Type I or Insulin Dependent is now correctly referred to as **Type 1**.

▶ Diabetes that was formerly referred to as Adult, Type II or Non-insulin Dependent is now correctly referred to as **Type 2**.

▶ There are other types under special medical circumstances. If your disease is not Type 1 or Type 2, then fill in your specific diagnosis.

PERSONAL INFORMATION

Name _____

Date of birth _____

Date first diagnosed with diabetes _____

Type 1 or 2 diabetes? (circle one) or List other type: _____

List **allergies** to medicines:_____

_____

_____

_____

Do you use **insulin** to control your diabetes? YES or NO

Current address: _____

_____

_____

_____

EMERGENCY NOTIFICATION:

Name _____

Address _____

_____

_____

Telephone number_____

PERSONAL PHYSICIAN: Name _____

Telephone number _____

MEDICAL AND SURGICAL HISTORY

▶ Fill in the information as directed. Just check mark the diseases that you have or have had. Leave the rest of the spaces blank. This will allow you to check mark additional diagnosis as they occur.

▶ While this section is designed to give your doctor the past medical history pertinent to your health care, space is left at the end of this section for additional history. You may also use this section to elaborate on the diagnosis you check. For example you may list the number and dates of each heart attack or your bypass operation or your stroke(s).

▶ Please keep this section as legible as possible. Clutter may lead to misinterpretation and compromise your medical outcome.

MEDICAL AND SURGICAL HISTORY

Tobacco: Currently smoke _____ packs of cigarettes per day.

Quit smoking in the year _____

I use other tobacco products. _____

I have never used tobacco products _____

I have _____ **alcoholic** drinks per DAY / WEEK / OCCASIONAL.

Check all diagnosis that apply:

Stroke....................................._____

Seizures ...._____

Cataracts ...._____

Heart disease ...._____

Heart attack ...._____

Asthma...................................._____

Heart burn (GERD)..................._____

Kidney disease.........................._____

Diabetic foot disease.................._____

High blood pressure ...._____

Claudication ...._____

Deep vein thrombosis................_____

No. of pregnancies...................._____

No. of deliveries ...._____

Mini-strokes (TIA)......................_____

Retinopathy ...._____

Macular degeneration................._____

Angina ...._____

Heart failure.............................._____

COPD ...._____

Peptic ulcer..............................._____

Claudication ...._____

Neuropathy................................_____

Obesity ...._____

Heart disease ...._____

Diverticulitis ...._____

Cancer ...._____

SURGICAL HISTORY

Check all procedures that apply:

Appendectomy ...._____

Gall bladder....................._____

Cataract..........................._____

Colonoscopy...................._____

Upper endoscopy (EGD)._____

Cesarean section ...._____

Heart bypass ...._____
Cardiac angiography ...._____
Angioplasty (balloon) ...._____
Stent placement ...._____
Tonsillectomy ...._____
Hysterectomy ...._____

List other diseases, hospitalizations and operations: _____

_____

_____

_____

_____

_____

_____

_____

_____

_____

_____

CURRENT MEDICATIONS

▶ List the names of your medications, dosage and times of day taken. If you take different doses of the same medication at different times, feel free to list these on separate lines. Again, legibility counts.

▶ In the insulin section fill in only those that apply and leave the rest blank. For specialized regimens, sliding scale regimens and insulin pump settings be as exact and legible as possible; giving type of insulin and when administered.

▶ Generally a diabetic should be on medications to control blood sugar, a daily aspirin, lipid controlling medications and possibly blood pressure medications with special preference towards medications called angiotensin converting enzyme (ACE) inhibitors for renal (kidney) protection.

CURRENT MEDICATIONS

Name of Medicine	Dosage	Taken Times Daily
_____	_____	_____
_____	_____	_____
_____	_____	_____
_____	_____	_____
_____	_____	_____
_____	_____	_____
_____	_____	_____
_____	_____	_____
_____	_____	_____
_____	_____	_____
_____	_____	_____
_____	_____	_____
_____	_____	_____

Name of **INSULIN** used: _____

Regular	Morning units _____	Evening units _____
NPH (lente)	Morning units _____	Evening units _____
Ultra Lente	Morning units _____	Evening units _____
70/30	Morning units _____	Evening units _____

Insulin pump settings: _____

_____

_____

_____

Sliding scale and specialized regimens: _____

_____

_____

_____

_____

_____

_____

_____

_____

_____

_____

_____

_____

_____

IMMUNIZATIONS

▶ Enter the dates for your most recent vaccination(s).
▶ Diabetics are considered to have impaired immune function. Therefore, they may have worse cases of infectious diseases, making them sicker and increasing likelihood of death. Immunizations play an important role in diabetic management.
▶ At a minimum diabetics should have:
   1) An annual influenza vaccination.
   2) One lifetime pneumococcus vaccination.
   3) Current tetanus vaccination.

Influenza

▶ Vaccinate annually. Each year 20 million Americans catch the flu and 20,000 of them die!

▶ All diabetic patients should receive an annual influenza vaccine beginning each September. Contra-indications include allergy to egg products or other components of the influenza vaccine and Guillain-Barré syndrome within 6 weeks of a previous influenza vaccination. The vaccination cannot cause influenza or other respiratory diseases. The most common side effect is soreness at the injection site.

▶ Prophylaxis with anti-influenza drugs such as Symmetrel (amantadine) and Flumadine (rimantadine) may be used if allergy prevents immunization. These drugs are effective only against Influenza A. The Food and Drug Administration (FDA) recently approved the use of Tamiflu (oseltamivir) prophylaxis. To date Relenza (zanamivir) is only approved for treatment of influenza infections, but presumably would be effective as an influenza prophylactic. Tamiflu and Relenza are effective against both Influenza A & B.

▶ *Influenza vaccination does not guarantee that one will not catch the flu!*
  1. The trivalent vaccine is constituted of strains of Influenza A & B most likely to circulate in the USA during influenza season. Exposure to another strain of influenza might result in infection.
  2. A vaccinated patient may become infected with a strain immunized against, but the disease should not be as severe.
  3. Many other viruses cause influenza-like symptoms, but are generally referred to as "the flu."

Influenza vaccination date   _____/_____/_____

Pneumococcus

▶ A.K.A. Streptococcus pneumoniae. One time vaccination.
▶ All diabetics should receive at least one pneumococcal vaccination. Indications for repeat vaccination include:
1. Patients over the age of 65 that were less than 65 years old at the time of their initial vaccination *and* more than 5 years have elapsed since their initial vaccination.
2. Other indications for repeat vaccination may include nephrotic syndrome, chronic renal disease and immunocompromised states.
▶ Up to half of patients receiving pneumococcal vaccination experience soreness at the injection site. Severe reactions are rare.
▶ It is well established that the pneumococcal vaccine is effective in reducing life threatening disease due to pneumococcal blood infection (pneumococcal bacteremia). Its effectiveness in preventing other pneumococcal disease remains uncertain, including pneumococcal pneumonia. One should also remember that other bacteria and viruses can cause pneumonia. *It is therefore a misnomer to refer to this vaccination as the "pneumonia shot!"*

Pneumococcal vaccination date #1 _____/_____/_____

#2 _____/_____/_____

Tetanus

▶ Boost every 10 years. Complete series may be indicated.
▶ Diphtheria-tetanus toxoid should be administered every 10 years. If over 30 years have elapsed or if one has never been immunized, the whole series should be administered. Contra-indications to tetanus vaccination include allergy to any component of the vaccine.

Tetanus vaccination date #1 _____/_____/_____

#2 _____/_____/_____

#3 _____/_____/_____

HOME BLOOD SUGAR MONITORING RECORDS

▶ Enter the times blood sugars were tested and the corresponding values.

▶ Goal values (approximate):
   1. **Fasting =100 mg/dL.** Usually first morning. No food or drink for $\geq$ 8 hours
   2. **Bedtime = 140 mg/dL.**
   3. **After meal = 140 mg/dL.** Two hours after meals.

▶ There is some debate as to how often Type 2 diabetics should monitor their blood sugars, but when doing so, a minimum of a fasting (morning) and bedtime measurement should be obtained. Since Type 2 diabetes tends to be a progressive disease needing medication changes, routine monitoring is required. Consult your physician for recommendations specific to your case. Type 2 diabetics that have become insulin requiring may require more frequent monitoring.

▶ Type 1 diabetics should check their sugars as prescribed by your physician to fit your insulin regimen. Generally, Type 1 diabetics should measure their blood sugars 3 or 4 times daily.

HOME BLOOD SUGAR MONITORING RECORDS

January

Goals:

Morning (fasting) approximately = 100

Bedtime approximately = 140

After meals (2 hours) approximately = 140

Monday, January 1:

Time: _____   Blood Sugar: _____

Time: _____   Blood Sugar: _____

Time: _____   Blood Sugar: _____

Time: _____   Blood Sugar: _____

Tuesday, January 2:

Time: _____   Blood Sugar: _____

Time: _____   Blood Sugar: _____

Time: _____   Blood Sugar: _____

Time: _____   Blood Sugar: _____

Wednesday, January 3:

Time: _____   Blood Sugar: _____

Time: _____   Blood Sugar: _____

Time: _____   Blood Sugar: _____

Time: _____   Blood Sugar: _____

Thursday, January 4:

Time: _____   Blood Sugar: _____

Time: _____   Blood Sugar: _____

Time: _____   Blood Sugar: _____

Time: _____   Blood Sugar: _____

Friday, January 5:

Time: _____   Blood Sugar: _____

Time: _____   Blood Sugar: _____

Time: _____   Blood Sugar: _____

Time: _____   Blood Sugar: _____

Saturday, January 6:

Time: _____   Blood Sugar: _____

Time: _____   Blood Sugar: _____

Time: _____   Blood Sugar: _____

Time: _____   Blood Sugar: _____

Sunday, January 7:

Time: _____   Blood Sugar: _____

Time: _____   Blood Sugar: _____

Time: _____   Blood Sugar: _____

Time: _____   Blood Sugar: _____

Monday, January 8:

Time: _____   Blood Sugar: _____

Time: _____   Blood Sugar: _____

Time: _____   Blood Sugar: _____

Time: _____   Blood Sugar: _____

Tuesday, January 9:

Time: _____   Blood Sugar: _____

Time: _____   Blood Sugar: _____

Time: _____   Blood Sugar: _____

Time: _____   Blood Sugar: _____

Wednesday, January 10:

Time: _____   Blood Sugar: _____

Time: _____   Blood Sugar: _____

Time: _____   Blood Sugar: _____

Time: _____   Blood Sugar: _____

Thursday, January 11:

Time: _____   Blood Sugar: _____

Time: _____   Blood Sugar: _____

Time: _____   Blood Sugar: _____

Time: _____   Blood Sugar: _____

Friday, January 12:

Time: _____   Blood Sugar: _____

Time: _____   Blood Sugar: _____

Time: _____   Blood Sugar: _____

Time: _____   Blood Sugar: _____

Saturday, January 13:

Time: _____   Blood Sugar: _____

Time: _____   Blood Sugar: _____

Time: _____   Blood Sugar: _____

Time: _____   Blood Sugar: _____

Sunday, January 14:

Time: _____   Blood Sugar: _____

Time: _____   Blood Sugar: _____

Time: _____   Blood Sugar: _____

Time: _____   Blood Sugar: _____

Monday, January 15:

Time: _____　　　　Blood Sugar: _____

Time: _____　　　　Blood Sugar: _____

Time: _____　　　　Blood Sugar: _____

Time: _____　　　　Blood Sugar: _____

Tuesday, January 16:

Time: _____　　　　Blood Sugar: _____

Time: _____　　　　Blood Sugar: _____

Time: _____　　　　Blood Sugar: _____

Time: _____　　　　Blood Sugar: _____

Wednesday, January 17:

Time: _____　　　　Blood Sugar: _____

Time: _____　　　　Blood Sugar: _____

Time: _____　　　　Blood Sugar: _____

Time: _____　　　　Blood Sugar: _____

Thursday, January 18:

Time: _____　　　　Blood Sugar: _____

Time: _____　　　　Blood Sugar: _____

Time: _____　　　　Blood Sugar: _____

Time: _____　　　　Blood Sugar: _____

Friday, January 19:

Time: _____　　　　Blood Sugar: _____

Time: _____　　　　Blood Sugar: _____

Time: _____　　　　Blood Sugar: _____

Time: _____　　　　Blood Sugar: _____

Saturday, January 20:

Time: _____   Blood Sugar: _____

Time: _____   Blood Sugar: _____

Time: _____   Blood Sugar: _____

Time: _____   Blood Sugar: _____

Sunday, January 21:

Time: _____   Blood Sugar: _____

Time: _____   Blood Sugar: _____

Time: _____   Blood Sugar: _____

Time: _____   Blood Sugar: _____

Monday, January 22:

Time: _____   Blood Sugar: _____

Time: _____   Blood Sugar: _____

Time: _____   Blood Sugar: _____

Time: _____   Blood Sugar: _____

Tuesday, January 23:

Time: _____   Blood Sugar: _____

Time: _____   Blood Sugar: _____

Time: _____   Blood Sugar: _____

Time: _____   Blood Sugar: _____

Wednesday, January 24:

Time: _____   Blood Sugar: _____

Time: _____   Blood Sugar: _____

Time: _____   Blood Sugar: _____

Time: _____   Blood Sugar: _____

Thursday, January 25:

Time: _____   Blood Sugar: _____

Time: _____   Blood Sugar: _____

Time: _____   Blood Sugar: _____

Time: _____   Blood Sugar: _____

Friday, January 26:

Time: _____   Blood Sugar: _____

Time: _____   Blood Sugar: _____

Time: _____   Blood Sugar: _____

Time: _____   Blood Sugar: _____

Saturday, January 27:

Time: _____ Blood Sugar: _____

Time: _____ Blood Sugar: _____

Time: _____ Blood Sugar: _____

Time: _____ Blood Sugar: _____

Sunday, January 28:

Time: _____ Blood Sugar: _____

Time: _____ Blood Sugar: _____

Time: _____ Blood Sugar: _____

Time: _____ Blood Sugar: _____

HOME BLOOD SUGAR MONITORING RECORDS

February

Goals:

Morning (fasting) approximately = 100

Bedtime approximately = 140

After meals (2 hours) approximately = 140

Monday, January 29:

Time: _____   Blood Sugar: _____

Time: _____   Blood Sugar: _____

Time: _____   Blood Sugar: _____

Time: _____   Blood Sugar: _____

Tuesday, January 30:

Time: _____   Blood Sugar: _____

Time: _____   Blood Sugar: _____

Time: _____   Blood Sugar: _____

Time: _____   Blood Sugar: _____

Wednesday, January 31:

Time: _____   Blood Sugar: _____

Time: _____   Blood Sugar: _____

Time: _____   Blood Sugar: _____

Time: _____   Blood Sugar: _____

Thursday, February 1:

Time: _____   Blood Sugar: _____

Time: _____   Blood Sugar: _____

Time: _____   Blood Sugar: _____

Time: _____   Blood Sugar: _____

Friday, February 2:

Time: _____   Blood Sugar: _____

Time: _____   Blood Sugar: _____

Time: _____   Blood Sugar: _____

Time: _____   Blood Sugar: _____

Saturday, February 3:

Time: _____   Blood Sugar: _____

Time: _____   Blood Sugar: _____

Time: _____   Blood Sugar: _____

Time: _____   Blood Sugar: _____

Sunday, February 4:

Time: _____   Blood Sugar: _____

Time: _____   Blood Sugar: _____

Time: _____   Blood Sugar: _____

Time: _____   Blood Sugar: _____

Monday, February 5:

Time: _____   Blood Sugar: _____

Time: _____   Blood Sugar: _____

Time: _____   Blood Sugar: _____

Time: _____   Blood Sugar: _____

Tuesday, February 6:

Time: _____   Blood Sugar: _____

Time: _____   Blood Sugar: _____

Time: _____   Blood Sugar: _____

Time: _____   Blood Sugar: _____

Wednesday, February 7:

Time: _____   Blood Sugar: _____

Time: _____   Blood Sugar: _____

Time: _____   Blood Sugar: _____

Time: _____   Blood Sugar: _____

Thursday, February 8:

Time: _____   Blood Sugar: _____

Time: _____   Blood Sugar: _____

Time: _____   Blood Sugar: _____

Time: _____   Blood Sugar: _____

Friday, February 9:

Time: _____   Blood Sugar: _____

Time: _____   Blood Sugar: _____

Time: _____   Blood Sugar: _____

Time: _____   Blood Sugar: _____

Saturday, February 10:

Time: _____   Blood Sugar: _____

Time: _____   Blood Sugar: _____

Time: _____   Blood Sugar: _____

Time: _____   Blood Sugar: _____

Sunday, February 11:

Time: _____   Blood Sugar: _____

Time: _____   Blood Sugar: _____

Time: _____   Blood Sugar: _____

Time: _____   Blood Sugar: _____

Monday, February 12:

Time: _____   Blood Sugar: _____

Time: _____   Blood Sugar: _____

Time: _____   Blood Sugar: _____

Time: _____   Blood Sugar: _____

Tuesday, February 13:

Time: _____   Blood Sugar: _____

Time: _____   Blood Sugar: _____

Time: _____   Blood Sugar: _____

Time: _____   Blood Sugar: _____

Wednesday, February 14:

Time: _____   Blood Sugar: _____

Time: _____   Blood Sugar: _____

Time: _____   Blood Sugar: _____

Time: _____   Blood Sugar: _____

Thursday, February 15:

Time: _____   Blood Sugar: _____

Time: _____   Blood Sugar: _____

Time: _____   Blood Sugar: _____

Time: _____   Blood Sugar: _____

Friday, February 16:

Time: _____   Blood Sugar: _____

Time: _____   Blood Sugar: _____

Time: _____   Blood Sugar: _____

Time: _____   Blood Sugar: _____

Saturday, February 17:

Time: _____   Blood Sugar: _____

Time: _____   Blood Sugar: _____

Time: _____   Blood Sugar: _____

Time: _____   Blood Sugar: _____

Sunday, February 18:

Time: _____   Blood Sugar: _____

Time: _____   Blood Sugar: _____

Time: _____   Blood Sugar: _____

Time: _____   Blood Sugar: _____

Monday, February 19:

Time: _____   Blood Sugar: _____

Time: _____   Blood Sugar: _____

Time: _____   Blood Sugar: _____

Time: _____   Blood Sugar: _____

Tuesday, February 20:

Time: _____   Blood Sugar: _____

Time: _____   Blood Sugar: _____

Time: _____   Blood Sugar: _____

Time: _____   Blood Sugar: _____

Wednesday, February 21:

Time: _____   Blood Sugar: _____

Time: _____   Blood Sugar: _____

Time: _____   Blood Sugar: _____

Time: _____   Blood Sugar: _____

Thursday, February 22:

Time: _____   Blood Sugar: _____

Time: _____   Blood Sugar: _____

Time: _____   Blood Sugar: _____

Time: _____   Blood Sugar: _____

Friday, February 23:

Time: _____   Blood Sugar: _____

Time: _____   Blood Sugar: _____

Time: _____   Blood Sugar: _____

Time: _____   Blood Sugar: _____

Saturday, February 24:

Time: _____ Blood Sugar: _____

Time: _____ Blood Sugar: _____

Time: _____ Blood Sugar: _____

Time: _____ Blood Sugar: _____

Sunday, February 25:

Time: _____ Blood Sugar: _____

Time: _____ Blood Sugar: _____

Time: _____ Blood Sugar: _____

Time: _____ Blood Sugar: _____

Home Blood Sugar Monitoring Records

March

Goals:

Morning (fasting) approximately = 100

Bedtime approximately = 140

After meals (2 hours) approximately = 140

Monday, February 26:

Time: _____   Blood Sugar: _____

Time: _____   Blood Sugar: _____

Time: _____   Blood Sugar: _____

Time: _____   Blood Sugar: _____

Tuesday, February 27:

Time: _____   Blood Sugar: _____

Time: _____   Blood Sugar: _____

Time: _____   Blood Sugar: _____

Time: _____   Blood Sugar: _____

Wednesday, February 28:

Time: _____   Blood Sugar: _____

Time: _____   Blood Sugar: _____

Time: _____   Blood Sugar: _____

Time: _____   Blood Sugar: _____

Thursday, March 1:

Time: _____   Blood Sugar: _____

Time: _____   Blood Sugar: _____

Time: _____   Blood Sugar: _____

Time: _____   Blood Sugar: _____

Friday, March 2:

Time: _____   Blood Sugar: _____

Time: _____   Blood Sugar: _____

Time: _____   Blood Sugar: _____

Time: _____   Blood Sugar: _____

Saturday, March 3:

Time: _____   Blood Sugar: _____

Time: _____   Blood Sugar: _____

Time: _____   Blood Sugar: _____

Time: _____   Blood Sugar: _____

Sunday, March 4:

Time: _____   Blood Sugar: _____

Time: _____   Blood Sugar: _____

Time: _____   Blood Sugar: _____

Time: _____   Blood Sugar: _____

Monday, March 5:

Time: _____   Blood Sugar: _____

Time: _____   Blood Sugar: _____

Time: _____   Blood Sugar: _____

Time: _____   Blood Sugar: _____

Tuesday, March 6:

Time: _____   Blood Sugar: _____

Time: _____   Blood Sugar: _____

Time: _____   Blood Sugar: _____

Time: _____   Blood Sugar: _____

Wednesday, March 7:

Time: _____   Blood Sugar: _____

Time: _____   Blood Sugar: _____

Time: _____   Blood Sugar: _____

Time: _____   Blood Sugar: _____

Thursday, March 8:

Time: _____   Blood Sugar: _____

Time: _____   Blood Sugar: _____

Time: _____   Blood Sugar: _____

Time: _____   Blood Sugar: _____

Friday, March 9:

Time: _____   Blood Sugar: _____

Time: _____   Blood Sugar: _____

Time: _____   Blood Sugar: _____

Time: _____   Blood Sugar: _____

Saturday, March 10:

Time: _____ Blood Sugar: _____

Time: _____ Blood Sugar: _____

Time: _____ Blood Sugar: _____

Time: _____ Blood Sugar: _____

Sunday, March 11:

Time: _____ Blood Sugar: _____

Time: _____ Blood Sugar: _____

Time: _____ Blood Sugar: _____

Time: _____ Blood Sugar: _____

Monday, March 12:

Time: _____   Blood Sugar: _____

Time: _____   Blood Sugar: _____

Time: _____   Blood Sugar: _____

Time: _____   Blood Sugar: _____

Tuesday, March 13:

Time: _____   Blood Sugar: _____

Time: _____   Blood Sugar: _____

Time: _____   Blood Sugar: _____

Time: _____   Blood Sugar: _____

Wednesday, March 14:

Time: _____   Blood Sugar: _____

Time: _____   Blood Sugar: _____

Time: _____   Blood Sugar: _____

Time: _____   Blood Sugar: _____

Thursday, March 15:

Time: _____   Blood Sugar: _____

Time: _____   Blood Sugar: _____

Time: _____   Blood Sugar: _____

Time: _____   Blood Sugar: _____

Friday, March 16:

Time: _____   Blood Sugar: _____

Time: _____   Blood Sugar: _____

Time: _____   Blood Sugar: _____

Time: _____   Blood Sugar: _____

Saturday, March 17:

Time: _____	Blood Sugar: _____
Time: _____	Blood Sugar: _____
Time: _____	Blood Sugar: _____
Time: _____	Blood Sugar: _____

Sunday, March 18:

Time: _____	Blood Sugar: _____
Time: _____	Blood Sugar: _____
Time: _____	Blood Sugar: _____
Time: _____	Blood Sugar: _____

Monday, March 19:

Time: _____   Blood Sugar: _____

Time: _____   Blood Sugar: _____

Time: _____   Blood Sugar: _____

Time: _____   Blood Sugar: _____

Tuesday, March 20:

Time: _____   Blood Sugar: _____

Time: _____   Blood Sugar: _____

Time: _____   Blood Sugar: _____

Time: _____   Blood Sugar: _____

Wednesday, March 21:

Time: _____   Blood Sugar: _____

Time: _____   Blood Sugar: _____

Time: _____   Blood Sugar: _____

Time: _____   Blood Sugar: _____

Thursday, March 22:

Time: _____   Blood Sugar: _____

Time: _____   Blood Sugar: _____

Time: _____   Blood Sugar: _____

Time: _____   Blood Sugar: _____

Friday, March 23:

Time: _____   Blood Sugar: _____

Time: _____   Blood Sugar: _____

Time: _____   Blood Sugar: _____

Time: _____   Blood Sugar: _____

Saturday, March 24:

Time: _____   Blood Sugar: _____

Time: _____   Blood Sugar: _____

Time: _____   Blood Sugar: _____

Time: _____   Blood Sugar: _____

Sunday, March 25:

Time: _____   Blood Sugar: _____

Time: _____   Blood Sugar: _____

Time: _____   Blood Sugar: _____

Time: _____   Blood Sugar: _____

Monday, March 26:

Time: _____   Blood Sugar: _____

Time: _____   Blood Sugar: _____

Time: _____   Blood Sugar: _____

Time: _____   Blood Sugar: _____

Tuesday, March 27:

Time: _____   Blood Sugar: _____

Time: _____   Blood Sugar: _____

Time: _____   Blood Sugar: _____

Time: _____   Blood Sugar: _____

Wednesday, March 28:

Time: _____   Blood Sugar: _____

Time: _____   Blood Sugar: _____

Time: _____   Blood Sugar: _____

Time: _____   Blood Sugar: _____

Thursday, March 29:

Time: _____   Blood Sugar: _____

Time: _____   Blood Sugar: _____

Time: _____   Blood Sugar: _____

Time: _____   Blood Sugar: _____

Friday, March 30:

Time: _____   Blood Sugar: _____

Time: _____   Blood Sugar: _____

Time: _____   Blood Sugar: _____

Time: _____   Blood Sugar: _____

Saturday, March 31:

Time: _____ Blood Sugar: _____

Time: _____ Blood Sugar: _____

Time: _____ Blood Sugar: _____

Time: _____ Blood Sugar: _____

Sunday, April 1:

Time: _____ Blood Sugar: _____

Time: _____ Blood Sugar: _____

Time: _____ Blood Sugar: _____

Time: _____ Blood Sugar: _____

HOME BLOOD SUGAR
MONITORING RECORDS

April

Goals: Morning (fasting) approximately = 100

Bedtime approximately = 140

After meals (2 hours) approximately = 140

Monday, April 2:

Time: _____   Blood Sugar: _____

Time: _____   Blood Sugar: _____

Time: _____   Blood Sugar: _____

Time: _____   Blood Sugar: _____

Tuesday, April 3:

Time: _____   Blood Sugar: _____

Time: _____   Blood Sugar: _____

Time: _____   Blood Sugar: _____

Time: _____   Blood Sugar: _____

Wednesday, April 4:

Time: _____   Blood Sugar: _____

Time: _____   Blood Sugar: _____

Time: _____   Blood Sugar: _____

Time: _____   Blood Sugar: _____

Thursday, April 5:

Time: _____   Blood Sugar: _____

Time: _____   Blood Sugar: _____

Time: _____   Blood Sugar: _____

Time: _____   Blood Sugar: _____

Friday, April 6:

Time: _____   Blood Sugar: _____

Time: _____   Blood Sugar: _____

Time: _____   Blood Sugar: _____

Time: _____   Blood Sugar: _____

Saturday, April 7:

Time: _____   Blood Sugar: _____

Time: _____   Blood Sugar: _____

Time: _____   Blood Sugar: _____

Time: _____   Blood Sugar: _____

Sunday, April 8:

Time: _____   Blood Sugar: _____

Time: _____   Blood Sugar: _____

Time: _____   Blood Sugar: _____

Time: _____   Blood Sugar: _____

Monday, April 9:

Time: _____   Blood Sugar: _____

Time: _____   Blood Sugar: _____

Time: _____   Blood Sugar: _____

Time: _____   Blood Sugar: _____

Tuesday, April 10:

Time: _____   Blood Sugar: _____

Time: _____   Blood Sugar: _____

Time: _____   Blood Sugar: _____

Time: _____   Blood Sugar: _____

Wednesday, April 11:

Time: _____   Blood Sugar: _____

Time: _____   Blood Sugar: _____

Time: _____   Blood Sugar: _____

Time: _____   Blood Sugar: _____

Thursday, April 12:

Time: _____   Blood Sugar: _____

Time: _____   Blood Sugar: _____

Time: _____   Blood Sugar: _____

Time: _____   Blood Sugar: _____

Friday, April 13:

Time: _____   Blood Sugar: _____

Time: _____   Blood Sugar: _____

Time: _____   Blood Sugar: _____

Time: _____   Blood Sugar: _____

Saturday, April 14:

Time: _____   Blood Sugar: _____

Time: _____   Blood Sugar: _____

Time: _____   Blood Sugar: _____

Time: _____   Blood Sugar: _____

Sunday, April 15:

Time: _____   Blood Sugar: _____

Time: _____   Blood Sugar: _____

Time: _____   Blood Sugar: _____

Time: _____   Blood Sugar: _____

Monday, April 16:

Time: _____   Blood Sugar: _____

Time: _____   Blood Sugar: _____

Time: _____   Blood Sugar: _____

Time: _____   Blood Sugar: _____

Tuesday, April 17:

Time: _____   Blood Sugar: _____

Time: _____   Blood Sugar: _____

Time: _____   Blood Sugar: _____

Time: _____   Blood Sugar: _____

Wednesday, April 18:

Time: _____   Blood Sugar: _____

Time: _____   Blood Sugar: _____

Time: _____   Blood Sugar: _____

Time: _____   Blood Sugar: _____

Thursday, April 19:

Time: _____   Blood Sugar: _____

Time: _____   Blood Sugar: _____

Time: _____   Blood Sugar: _____

Time: _____   Blood Sugar: _____

Friday, April 20:

Time: _____   Blood Sugar: _____

Time: _____   Blood Sugar: _____

Time: _____   Blood Sugar: _____

Time: _____   Blood Sugar: _____

Saturday, April 21:

Time: _____   Blood Sugar: _____

Time: _____   Blood Sugar: _____

Time: _____   Blood Sugar: _____

Time: _____   Blood Sugar: _____

Sunday, April 22:

Time: _____   Blood Sugar: _____

Time: _____   Blood Sugar: _____

Time: _____   Blood Sugar: _____

Time: _____   Blood Sugar: _____

Monday, April 23:

Time: _____   Blood Sugar: _____

Time: _____   Blood Sugar: _____

Time: _____   Blood Sugar: _____

Time: _____   Blood Sugar: _____

Tuesday, April 24:

Time: _____   Blood Sugar: _____

Time: _____   Blood Sugar: _____

Time: _____   Blood Sugar: _____

Time: _____   Blood Sugar: _____

Wednesday, April 25:

Time: _____   Blood Sugar: _____

Time: _____   Blood Sugar: _____

Time: _____   Blood Sugar: _____

Time: _____   Blood Sugar: _____

Thursday, April 26:

Time: _____   Blood Sugar: _____

Time: _____   Blood Sugar: _____

Time: _____   Blood Sugar: _____

Time: _____   Blood Sugar: _____

Friday, April 27:

Time: _____   Blood Sugar: _____

Time: _____   Blood Sugar: _____

Time: _____   Blood Sugar: _____

Time: _____   Blood Sugar: _____

Saturday, April 28:

Time: _____ Blood Sugar: _____

Time: _____ Blood Sugar: _____

Time: _____ Blood Sugar: _____

Time: _____ Blood Sugar: _____

Sunday, April 29:

Time: _____ Blood Sugar: _____

Time: _____ Blood Sugar: _____

Time: _____ Blood Sugar: _____

Time: _____ Blood Sugar: _____

Home Blood Sugar Monitoring Records

May

Goals:

Morning (fasting) approximately = 100

Bedtime approximately = 140

After meals (2 hours) approximately = 140

Monday, April 30:

Time: _____   Blood Sugar: _____

Time: _____   Blood Sugar: _____

Time: _____   Blood Sugar: _____

Time: _____   Blood Sugar: _____

Tuesday, May 1:

Time: _____   Blood Sugar: _____

Time: _____   Blood Sugar: _____

Time: _____   Blood Sugar: _____

Time: _____   Blood Sugar: _____

Wednesday, May 2:

Time: _____   Blood Sugar: _____

Time: _____   Blood Sugar: _____

Time: _____   Blood Sugar: _____

Time: _____   Blood Sugar: _____

Thursday, May 3:

Time: _____   Blood Sugar: _____

Time: _____   Blood Sugar: _____

Time: _____   Blood Sugar: _____

Time: _____   Blood Sugar: _____

Friday, May 4:

Time: _____   Blood Sugar: _____

Time: _____   Blood Sugar: _____

Time: _____   Blood Sugar: _____

Time: _____   Blood Sugar: _____

Saturday, May 5:

Time: _____ Blood Sugar: _____

Time: _____ Blood Sugar: _____

Time: _____ Blood Sugar: _____

Time: _____ Blood Sugar: _____

Sunday, May 6:

Time: _____ Blood Sugar: _____

Time: _____ Blood Sugar: _____

Time: _____ Blood Sugar: _____

Time: _____ Blood Sugar: _____

Monday, May 7:

Time: _____   Blood Sugar: _____

Time: _____   Blood Sugar: _____

Time: _____   Blood Sugar: _____

Time: _____   Blood Sugar: _____

Tuesday, May 8:

Time: _____   Blood Sugar: _____

Time: _____   Blood Sugar: _____

Time: _____   Blood Sugar: _____

Time: _____   Blood Sugar: _____

Wednesday, May 9:

Time: _____   Blood Sugar: _____

Time: _____   Blood Sugar: _____

Time: _____   Blood Sugar: _____

Time: _____   Blood Sugar: _____

Thursday, May 10:

Time: _____   Blood Sugar: _____

Time: _____   Blood Sugar: _____

Time: _____   Blood Sugar: _____

Time: _____   Blood Sugar: _____

Friday, May 11:

Time: _____   Blood Sugar: _____

Time: _____   Blood Sugar: _____

Time: _____   Blood Sugar: _____

Time: _____   Blood Sugar: _____

Saturday, May 12:

Time: _____   Blood Sugar: _____

Time: _____   Blood Sugar: _____

Time: _____   Blood Sugar: _____

Time: _____   Blood Sugar: _____

Sunday, May 13:

Time: _____   Blood Sugar: _____

Time: _____   Blood Sugar: _____

Time: _____   Blood Sugar: _____

Time: _____   Blood Sugar: _____

Monday, May 14:

Time: _____   Blood Sugar: _____

Time: _____   Blood Sugar: _____

Time: _____   Blood Sugar: _____

Time: _____   Blood Sugar: _____

Tuesday, May 15:

Time: _____   Blood Sugar: _____

Time: _____   Blood Sugar: _____

Time: _____   Blood Sugar: _____

Time: _____   Blood Sugar: _____

Wednesday, May 16:

Time: _____   Blood Sugar: _____

Time: _____   Blood Sugar: _____

Time: _____   Blood Sugar: _____

Time: _____   Blood Sugar: _____

Thursday, May 17:

Time: _____   Blood Sugar: _____

Time: _____   Blood Sugar: _____

Time: _____   Blood Sugar: _____

Time: _____   Blood Sugar: _____

Friday, May 18:

Time: _____   Blood Sugar: _____

Time: _____   Blood Sugar: _____

Time: _____   Blood Sugar: _____

Time: _____   Blood Sugar: _____

Saturday, May 19:

Time: _____   Blood Sugar: _____

Time: _____   Blood Sugar: _____

Time: _____   Blood Sugar: _____

Time: _____   Blood Sugar: _____

Sunday, May 20:

Time: _____   Blood Sugar: _____

Time: _____   Blood Sugar: _____

Time: _____   Blood Sugar: _____

Time: _____   Blood Sugar: _____

Monday, May 21:

Time: _____   Blood Sugar: _____

Time: _____   Blood Sugar: _____

Time: _____   Blood Sugar: _____

Time: _____   Blood Sugar: _____

Tuesday, May 22:

Time: _____   Blood Sugar: _____

Time: _____   Blood Sugar: _____

Time: _____   Blood Sugar: _____

Time: _____   Blood Sugar: _____

Wednesday, May 23:

Time: _____   Blood Sugar: _____

Time: _____   Blood Sugar: _____

Time: _____   Blood Sugar: _____

Time: _____   Blood Sugar: _____

Thursday, May 24:

Time: _____   Blood Sugar: _____

Time: _____   Blood Sugar: _____

Time: _____   Blood Sugar: _____

Time: _____   Blood Sugar: _____

Friday, May 25:

Time: _____   Blood Sugar: _____

Time: _____   Blood Sugar: _____

Time: _____   Blood Sugar: _____

Time: _____   Blood Sugar: _____

Saturday, May 26:

Time: _____ Blood Sugar: _____

Time: _____ Blood Sugar: _____

Time: _____ Blood Sugar: _____

Time: _____ Blood Sugar: _____

Sunday, May 27:

Time: _____ Blood Sugar: _____

Time: _____ Blood Sugar: _____

Time: _____ Blood Sugar: _____

Time: _____ Blood Sugar: _____

Home Blood Sugar Monitoring Records

June

Goals:

Morning (fasting) approximately = 100

Bedtime approximately = 140

After meals (2 hours) approximately = 140

Monday, May 28:

Time: _____   Blood Sugar: _____

Time: _____   Blood Sugar: _____

Time: _____   Blood Sugar: _____

Time: _____   Blood Sugar: _____

Tuesday, May 29:

Time: _____   Blood Sugar: _____

Time: _____   Blood Sugar: _____

Time: _____   Blood Sugar: _____

Time: _____   Blood Sugar: _____

Wednesday, May 30:

Time: _____   Blood Sugar: _____

Time: _____   Blood Sugar: _____

Time: _____   Blood Sugar: _____

Time: _____   Blood Sugar: _____

Thursday, May 31:

Time: _____   Blood Sugar: _____

Time: _____   Blood Sugar: _____

Time: _____   Blood Sugar: _____

Time: _____   Blood Sugar: _____

Friday, June 1:

Time: _____   Blood Sugar: _____

Time: _____   Blood Sugar: _____

Time: _____   Blood Sugar: _____

Time: _____   Blood Sugar: _____

Saturday, June 2:

Time: _____   Blood Sugar: _____

Time: _____   Blood Sugar: _____

Time: _____   Blood Sugar: _____

Time: _____   Blood Sugar: _____

Sunday, June 3:

Time: _____   Blood Sugar: _____

Time: _____   Blood Sugar: _____

Time: _____   Blood Sugar: _____

Time: _____   Blood Sugar: _____

Monday, June 4:

Time: _____   Blood Sugar: _____

Time: _____   Blood Sugar: _____

Time: _____   Blood Sugar: _____

Time: _____   Blood Sugar: _____

Tuesday, June 5:

Time: _____   Blood Sugar: _____

Time: _____   Blood Sugar: _____

Time: _____   Blood Sugar: _____

Time: _____   Blood Sugar: _____

Wednesday, June 6:

Time: _____   Blood Sugar: _____

Time: _____   Blood Sugar: _____

Time: _____   Blood Sugar: _____

Time: _____   Blood Sugar: _____

Thursday, June 7:

Time: _____   Blood Sugar: _____

Time: _____   Blood Sugar: _____

Time: _____   Blood Sugar: _____

Time: _____   Blood Sugar: _____

Friday, June 8:

Time: _____   Blood Sugar: _____

Time: _____   Blood Sugar: _____

Time: _____   Blood Sugar: _____

Time: _____   Blood Sugar: _____

Saturday, June 9:

Time: _____   Blood Sugar: _____

Time: _____   Blood Sugar: _____

Time: _____   Blood Sugar: _____

Time: _____   Blood Sugar: _____

Sunday, June 10:

Time: _____   Blood Sugar: _____

Time: _____   Blood Sugar: _____

Time: _____   Blood Sugar: _____

Time: _____   Blood Sugar: _____

Monday, June 11:

Time: _____   Blood Sugar: _____

Time: _____   Blood Sugar: _____

Time: _____   Blood Sugar: _____

Time: _____   Blood Sugar: _____

Tuesday, June 12:

Time: _____   Blood Sugar: _____

Time: _____   Blood Sugar: _____

Time: _____   Blood Sugar: _____

Time: _____   Blood Sugar: _____

Wednesday, June 13:

Time: _____   Blood Sugar: _____

Time: _____   Blood Sugar: _____

Time: _____   Blood Sugar: _____

Time: _____   Blood Sugar: _____

Thursday, June 14:

Time: _____   Blood Sugar: _____

Time: _____   Blood Sugar: _____

Time: _____   Blood Sugar: _____

Time: _____   Blood Sugar: _____

Friday, June 15:

Time: _____   Blood Sugar: _____

Time: _____   Blood Sugar: _____

Time: _____   Blood Sugar: _____

Time: _____   Blood Sugar: _____

Saturday, June 16:

Time: _____   Blood Sugar: _____

Time: _____   Blood Sugar: _____

Time: _____   Blood Sugar: _____

Time: _____   Blood Sugar: _____

Sunday, June 17:

Time: _____   Blood Sugar: _____

Time: _____   Blood Sugar: _____

Time: _____   Blood Sugar: _____

Time: _____   Blood Sugar: _____

Monday, June 18:

Time: _____ Blood Sugar: _____

Time: _____ Blood Sugar: _____

Time: _____ Blood Sugar: _____

Time: _____ Blood Sugar: _____

Tuesday, June 19:

Time: _____ Blood Sugar: _____

Time: _____ Blood Sugar: _____

Time: _____ Blood Sugar: _____

Time: _____ Blood Sugar: _____

Wednesday, June 20:

Time: _____ Blood Sugar: _____

Time: _____ Blood Sugar: _____

Time: _____ Blood Sugar: _____

Time: _____ Blood Sugar: _____

Thursday, June 21:

Time: _____ Blood Sugar: _____

Time: _____ Blood Sugar: _____

Time: _____ Blood Sugar: _____

Time: _____ Blood Sugar: _____

Friday, June 22:

Time: _____ Blood Sugar: _____

Time: _____ Blood Sugar: _____

Time: _____ Blood Sugar: _____

Time: _____ Blood Sugar: _____

Saturday, June 23:

Time: _____   Blood Sugar: _____

Time: _____   Blood Sugar: _____

Time: _____   Blood Sugar: _____

Time: _____   Blood Sugar: _____

Sunday, June 24:

Time: _____   Blood Sugar: _____

Time: _____   Blood Sugar: _____

Time: _____   Blood Sugar: _____

Time: _____   Blood Sugar: _____

Monday, June 25:

Time: _____   Blood Sugar: _____

Time: _____   Blood Sugar: _____

Time: _____   Blood Sugar: _____

Time: _____   Blood Sugar: _____

Tuesday, June 26:

Time: _____   Blood Sugar: _____

Time: _____   Blood Sugar: _____

Time: _____   Blood Sugar: _____

Time: _____   Blood Sugar: _____

Wednesday, June 27:

Time: _____   Blood Sugar: _____

Time: _____   Blood Sugar: _____

Time: _____   Blood Sugar: _____

Time: _____   Blood Sugar: _____

Thursday, June 28:

Time: _____   Blood Sugar: _____

Time: _____   Blood Sugar: _____

Time: _____   Blood Sugar: _____

Time: _____   Blood Sugar: _____

Friday, June 29:

Time: _____   Blood Sugar: _____

Time: _____   Blood Sugar: _____

Time: _____   Blood Sugar: _____

Time: _____   Blood Sugar: _____

Saturday, June 30:

Time: _____ Blood Sugar: _____

Time: _____ Blood Sugar: _____

Time: _____ Blood Sugar: _____

Time: _____ Blood Sugar: _____

Sunday, July 1:

Time: _____ Blood Sugar: _____

Time: _____ Blood Sugar: _____

Time: _____ Blood Sugar: _____

Time: _____ Blood Sugar: _____

Home Blood Sugar
Monitoring Records

July

Goals:

Morning (fasting) approximately = 100

Bedtime approximately = 140

After meals (2 hours) approximately = 140

Monday, July 2:

Time: _____   Blood Sugar: _____

Time: _____   Blood Sugar: _____

Time: _____   Blood Sugar: _____

Time: _____   Blood Sugar: _____

Tuesday, July 3:

Time: _____   Blood Sugar: _____

Time: _____   Blood Sugar: _____

Time: _____   Blood Sugar: _____

Time: _____   Blood Sugar: _____

Wednesday, July 4:

Time: _____   Blood Sugar: _____

Time: _____   Blood Sugar: _____

Time: _____   Blood Sugar: _____

Time: _____   Blood Sugar: _____

Thursday, July 5:

Time: _____   Blood Sugar: _____

Time: _____   Blood Sugar: _____

Time: _____   Blood Sugar: _____

Time: _____   Blood Sugar: _____

Friday, July 6:

Time: _____   Blood Sugar: _____

Time: _____   Blood Sugar: _____

Time: _____   Blood Sugar: _____

Time: _____   Blood Sugar: _____

Saturday, July 7:

Time: _____   Blood Sugar: _____

Time: _____   Blood Sugar: _____

Time: _____   Blood Sugar: _____

Time: _____   Blood Sugar: _____

Sunday, July 8:

Time: _____   Blood Sugar: _____

Time: _____   Blood Sugar: _____

Time: _____   Blood Sugar: _____

Time: _____   Blood Sugar: _____

Monday, July 9:

Time: _____ Blood Sugar: _____

Time: _____ Blood Sugar: _____

Time: _____ Blood Sugar: _____

Time: _____ Blood Sugar: _____

Tuesday, July 10:

Time: _____ Blood Sugar: _____

Time: _____ Blood Sugar: _____

Time: _____ Blood Sugar: _____

Time: _____ Blood Sugar: _____

Wednesday, July 11:

Time: _____ Blood Sugar: _____

Time: _____ Blood Sugar: _____

Time: _____ Blood Sugar: _____

Time: _____ Blood Sugar: _____

Thursday, July 12:

Time: _____ Blood Sugar: _____

Time: _____ Blood Sugar: _____

Time: _____ Blood Sugar: _____

Time: _____ Blood Sugar: _____

Friday, July 13:

Time: _____ Blood Sugar: _____

Time: _____ Blood Sugar: _____

Time: _____ Blood Sugar: _____

Time: _____ Blood Sugar: _____

Saturday, July 14:

Time: _____   Blood Sugar: _____

Time: _____   Blood Sugar: _____

Time: _____   Blood Sugar: _____

Time: _____   Blood Sugar: _____

Sunday, July 15:

Time: _____   Blood Sugar: _____

Time: _____   Blood Sugar: _____

Time: _____   Blood Sugar: _____

Time: _____   Blood Sugar: _____

Monday, July 16:

Time: _____   Blood Sugar: _____

Time: _____   Blood Sugar: _____

Time: _____   Blood Sugar: _____

Time: _____   Blood Sugar: _____

Tuesday, July 17:

Time: _____   Blood Sugar: _____

Time: _____   Blood Sugar: _____

Time: _____   Blood Sugar: _____

Time: _____   Blood Sugar: _____

Wednesday, July 18:

Time: _____   Blood Sugar: _____

Time: _____   Blood Sugar: _____

Time: _____   Blood Sugar: _____

Time: _____   Blood Sugar: _____

Thursday, July 19:

Time: _____   Blood Sugar: _____

Time: _____   Blood Sugar: _____

Time: _____   Blood Sugar: _____

Time: _____   Blood Sugar: _____

Friday, July 20:

Time: _____   Blood Sugar: _____

Time: _____   Blood Sugar: _____

Time: _____   Blood Sugar: _____

Time: _____   Blood Sugar: _____

Saturday, July 21:

Time: _____   Blood Sugar: _____

Time: _____   Blood Sugar: _____

Time: _____   Blood Sugar: _____

Time: _____   Blood Sugar: _____

Sunday, July 22:

Time: _____   Blood Sugar: _____

Time: _____   Blood Sugar: _____

Time: _____   Blood Sugar: _____

Time: _____   Blood Sugar: _____

Monday, July 23:

Time: _____   Blood Sugar: _____

Time: _____   Blood Sugar: _____

Time: _____   Blood Sugar: _____

Time: _____   Blood Sugar: _____

Tuesday, July 24:

Time: _____   Blood Sugar: _____

Time: _____   Blood Sugar: _____

Time: _____   Blood Sugar: _____

Time: _____   Blood Sugar: _____

Wednesday, July 25:

Time: _____   Blood Sugar: _____

Time: _____   Blood Sugar: _____

Time: _____   Blood Sugar: _____

Time: _____   Blood Sugar: _____

Thursday, July 26:

Time: _____   Blood Sugar: _____

Time: _____   Blood Sugar: _____

Time: _____   Blood Sugar: _____

Time: _____   Blood Sugar: _____

Friday, July 27:

Time: _____   Blood Sugar: _____

Time: _____   Blood Sugar: _____

Time: _____   Blood Sugar: _____

Time: _____   Blood Sugar: _____

Saturday, July 28:

Time: _____ Blood Sugar: _____

Time: _____ Blood Sugar: _____

Time: _____ Blood Sugar: _____

Time: _____ Blood Sugar: _____

Sunday, July 29:

Time: _____ Blood Sugar: _____

Time: _____ Blood Sugar: _____

Time: _____ Blood Sugar: _____

Time: _____ Blood Sugar: _____

HOME BLOOD SUGAR
MONITORING RECORDS

August

Goals:

Morning (fasting) approximately = 100

Bedtime approximately = 140

After meals (2 hours) approximately = 140

Monday, July 30:

Time: _____   Blood Sugar: _____

Time: _____   Blood Sugar: _____

Time: _____   Blood Sugar: _____

Time: _____   Blood Sugar: _____

Tuesday, July 31:

Time: _____   Blood Sugar: _____

Time: _____   Blood Sugar: _____

Time: _____   Blood Sugar: _____

Time: _____   Blood Sugar: _____

Wednesday, August 1:

Time: _____   Blood Sugar: _____

Time: _____   Blood Sugar: _____

Time: _____   Blood Sugar: _____

Time: _____   Blood Sugar: _____

Thursday, August 2:

Time: _____   Blood Sugar: _____

Time: _____   Blood Sugar: _____

Time: _____   Blood Sugar: _____

Time: _____   Blood Sugar: _____

Friday, August 3:

Time: _____   Blood Sugar: _____

Time: _____   Blood Sugar: _____

Time: _____   Blood Sugar: _____

Time: _____   Blood Sugar: _____

Saturday, August 4:

Time: _____ Blood Sugar: _____

Time: _____ Blood Sugar: _____

Time: _____ Blood Sugar: _____

Time: _____ Blood Sugar: _____

Sunday, August 5:

Time: _____ Blood Sugar: _____

Time: _____ Blood Sugar: _____

Time: _____ Blood Sugar: _____

Time: _____ Blood Sugar: _____

Monday, August 6:

Time: _____   Blood Sugar: _____

Time: _____   Blood Sugar: _____

Time: _____   Blood Sugar: _____

Time: _____   Blood Sugar: _____

Tuesday, August 7:

Time: _____   Blood Sugar: _____

Time: _____   Blood Sugar: _____

Time: _____   Blood Sugar: _____

Time: _____   Blood Sugar: _____

Wednesday, August 8:

Time: _____   Blood Sugar: _____

Time: _____   Blood Sugar: _____

Time: _____   Blood Sugar: _____

Time: _____   Blood Sugar: _____

Thursday, August 9:

Time: _____   Blood Sugar: _____

Time: _____   Blood Sugar: _____

Time: _____   Blood Sugar: _____

Time: _____   Blood Sugar: _____

Friday, August 10:

Time: _____   Blood Sugar: _____

Time: _____   Blood Sugar: _____

Time: _____   Blood Sugar: _____

Time: _____   Blood Sugar: _____

Saturday, August 11:

Time: _____   Blood Sugar: _____

Time: _____   Blood Sugar: _____

Time: _____   Blood Sugar: _____

Time: _____   Blood Sugar: _____

Sunday, August 12:

Time: _____   Blood Sugar: _____

Time: _____   Blood Sugar: _____

Time: _____   Blood Sugar: _____

Time: _____   Blood Sugar: _____

Monday, August 13:

Time: _____   Blood Sugar: _____

Time: _____   Blood Sugar: _____

Time: _____   Blood Sugar: _____

Time: _____   Blood Sugar: _____

Tuesday, August 14:

Time: _____   Blood Sugar: _____

Time: _____   Blood Sugar: _____

Time: _____   Blood Sugar: _____

Time: _____   Blood Sugar: _____

Wednesday, August 15:

Time: _____   Blood Sugar: _____

Time: _____   Blood Sugar: _____

Time: _____   Blood Sugar: _____

Time: _____   Blood Sugar: _____

Thursday, August 16:

Time: _____   Blood Sugar: _____

Time: _____   Blood Sugar: _____

Time: _____   Blood Sugar: _____

Time: _____   Blood Sugar: _____

Friday, August 17:

Time: _____   Blood Sugar: _____

Time: _____   Blood Sugar: _____

Time: _____   Blood Sugar: _____

Time: _____   Blood Sugar: _____

Saturday, August 18:

Time: _____   Blood Sugar: _____

Time: _____   Blood Sugar: _____

Time: _____   Blood Sugar: _____

Time: _____   Blood Sugar: _____

Sunday, August 19:

Time: _____   Blood Sugar: _____

Time: _____   Blood Sugar: _____

Time: _____   Blood Sugar: _____

Time: _____   Blood Sugar: _____

Monday, August 20:

Time: _____   Blood Sugar: _____

Time: _____   Blood Sugar: _____

Time: _____   Blood Sugar: _____

Time: _____   Blood Sugar: _____

Tuesday, August 21:

Time: _____   Blood Sugar: _____

Time: _____   Blood Sugar: _____

Time: _____   Blood Sugar: _____

Time: _____   Blood Sugar: _____

Wednesday, August 22:

Time: _____   Blood Sugar: _____

Time: _____   Blood Sugar: _____

Time: _____   Blood Sugar: _____

Time: _____   Blood Sugar: _____

Thursday, August 23:

Time: _____   Blood Sugar: _____

Time: _____   Blood Sugar: _____

Time: _____   Blood Sugar: _____

Time: _____   Blood Sugar: _____

Friday, August 24:

Time: _____   Blood Sugar: _____

Time: _____   Blood Sugar: _____

Time: _____   Blood Sugar: _____

Time: _____   Blood Sugar: _____

Saturday, August 25:

Time: _____   Blood Sugar: _____

Time: _____   Blood Sugar: _____

Time: _____   Blood Sugar: _____

Time: _____   Blood Sugar: _____

Sunday, August 26:

Time: _____   Blood Sugar: _____

Time: _____   Blood Sugar: _____

Time: _____   Blood Sugar: _____

Time: _____   Blood Sugar: _____

Monday, August 27:

Time: _____   Blood Sugar: _____

Time: _____   Blood Sugar: _____

Time: _____   Blood Sugar: _____

Time: _____   Blood Sugar: _____

Tuesday, August 28:

Time: _____   Blood Sugar: _____

Time: _____   Blood Sugar: _____

Time: _____   Blood Sugar: _____

Time: _____   Blood Sugar: _____

Wednesday, August 29:

Time: _____   Blood Sugar: _____

Time: _____   Blood Sugar: _____

Time: _____   Blood Sugar: _____

Time: _____   Blood Sugar: _____

Thursday, August 30:

Time: _____   Blood Sugar: _____

Time: _____   Blood Sugar: _____

Time: _____   Blood Sugar: _____

Time: _____   Blood Sugar: _____

Friday, August 31:

Time: _____   Blood Sugar: _____

Time: _____   Blood Sugar: _____

Time: _____   Blood Sugar: _____

Time: _____   Blood Sugar: _____

Saturday, September 1:

Time: _____ Blood Sugar: _____

Time: _____ Blood Sugar: _____

Time: _____ Blood Sugar: _____

Time: _____ Blood Sugar: _____

Sunday, September 2:

Time: _____ Blood Sugar: _____

Time: _____ Blood Sugar: _____

Time: _____ Blood Sugar: _____

Time: _____ Blood Sugar: _____

HOME BLOOD SUGAR MONITORING RECORDS

September

Goals:

Morning (fasting) approximately = 100

Bedtime approximately = 140

After meals (2 hours) approximately = 140

Monday, September 3:

Time: _____   Blood Sugar: _____

Time: _____   Blood Sugar: _____

Time: _____   Blood Sugar: _____

Time: _____   Blood Sugar: _____

Tuesday, September 4:

Time: _____   Blood Sugar: _____

Time: _____   Blood Sugar: _____

Time: _____   Blood Sugar: _____

Time: _____   Blood Sugar: _____

Wednesday, September 5:

Time: _____   Blood Sugar: _____

Time: _____   Blood Sugar: _____

Time: _____   Blood Sugar: _____

Time: _____   Blood Sugar: _____

Thursday, September 6:

Time: _____   Blood Sugar: _____

Time: _____   Blood Sugar: _____

Time: _____   Blood Sugar: _____

Time: _____   Blood Sugar: _____

Friday, September 7:

Time: _____   Blood Sugar: _____

Time: _____   Blood Sugar: _____

Time: _____   Blood Sugar: _____

Time: _____   Blood Sugar: _____

Saturday, September 8:

Time: _____   Blood Sugar: _____

Time: _____   Blood Sugar: _____

Time: _____   Blood Sugar: _____

Time: _____   Blood Sugar: _____

Sunday, September 9:

Time: _____   Blood Sugar: _____

Time: _____   Blood Sugar: _____

Time: _____   Blood Sugar: _____

Time: _____   Blood Sugar: _____

Monday, September 10:

Time: _____   Blood Sugar: _____

Time: _____   Blood Sugar: _____

Time: _____   Blood Sugar: _____

Time: _____   Blood Sugar: _____

Tuesday, September 11:

Time: _____   Blood Sugar: _____

Time: _____   Blood Sugar: _____

Time: _____   Blood Sugar: _____

Time: _____   Blood Sugar: _____

Wednesday, September 12:

Time: _____   Blood Sugar: _____

Time: _____   Blood Sugar: _____

Time: _____   Blood Sugar: _____

Time: _____   Blood Sugar: _____

Thursday, September 13:

Time: _____   Blood Sugar: _____

Time: _____   Blood Sugar: _____

Time: _____   Blood Sugar: _____

Time: _____   Blood Sugar: _____

Friday, September 14:

Time: _____   Blood Sugar: _____

Time: _____   Blood Sugar: _____

Time: _____   Blood Sugar: _____

Time: _____   Blood Sugar: _____

Saturday, September 15:

Time: _____   Blood Sugar: _____

Time: _____   Blood Sugar: _____

Time: _____   Blood Sugar: _____

Time: _____   Blood Sugar: _____

Sunday, September 16:

Time: _____   Blood Sugar: _____

Time: _____   Blood Sugar: _____

Time: _____   Blood Sugar: _____

Time: _____   Blood Sugar: _____

Monday, September 17:

Time: _____   Blood Sugar: _____

Time: _____   Blood Sugar: _____

Time: _____   Blood Sugar: _____

Time: _____   Blood Sugar: _____

Tuesday, September 18:

Time: _____   Blood Sugar: _____

Time: _____   Blood Sugar: _____

Time: _____   Blood Sugar: _____

Time: _____   Blood Sugar: _____

Wednesday, September 19:

Time: _____   Blood Sugar: _____

Time: _____   Blood Sugar: _____

Time: _____   Blood Sugar: _____

Time: _____   Blood Sugar: _____

Thursday, September 20:

Time: _____   Blood Sugar: _____

Time: _____   Blood Sugar: _____

Time: _____   Blood Sugar: _____

Time: _____   Blood Sugar: _____

Friday, September 21:

Time: _____   Blood Sugar: _____

Time: _____   Blood Sugar: _____

Time: _____   Blood Sugar: _____

Time: _____   Blood Sugar: _____

Saturday, September 22:

Time: _____   Blood Sugar: _____

Time: _____   Blood Sugar: _____

Time: _____   Blood Sugar: _____

Time: _____   Blood Sugar: _____

Sunday, September 23:

Time: _____   Blood Sugar: _____

Time: _____   Blood Sugar: _____

Time: _____   Blood Sugar: _____

Time: _____   Blood Sugar: _____

Monday, September 24:

Time: _____   Blood Sugar: _____

Time: _____   Blood Sugar: _____

Time: _____   Blood Sugar: _____

Time: _____   Blood Sugar: _____

Tuesday, September 25:

Time: _____   Blood Sugar: _____

Time: _____   Blood Sugar: _____

Time: _____   Blood Sugar: _____

Time: _____   Blood Sugar: _____

Wednesday, September 26:

Time: _____   Blood Sugar: _____

Time: _____   Blood Sugar: _____

Time: _____   Blood Sugar: _____

Time: _____   Blood Sugar: _____

Thursday, September 27:

Time: _____   Blood Sugar: _____

Time: _____   Blood Sugar: _____

Time: _____   Blood Sugar: _____

Time: _____   Blood Sugar: _____

Friday, September 28:

Time: _____   Blood Sugar: _____

Time: _____   Blood Sugar: _____

Time: _____   Blood Sugar: _____

Time: _____   Blood Sugar: _____

Saturday, September 29:

Time: _____ Blood Sugar: _____

Time: _____ Blood Sugar: _____

Time: _____ Blood Sugar: _____

Time: _____ Blood Sugar: _____

Sunday, September 30:

Time: _____ Blood Sugar: _____

Time: _____ Blood Sugar: _____

Time: _____ Blood Sugar: _____

Time: _____ Blood Sugar: _____

HOME BLOOD SUGAR MONITORING RECORDS

October

Goals:

Morning (fasting) approximately = 100

Bedtime approximately = 140

After meals (2 hours) approximately = 140

Monday, October 1:

Time: _____   Blood Sugar: _____

Time: _____   Blood Sugar: _____

Time: _____   Blood Sugar: _____

Time: _____   Blood Sugar: _____

Tuesday, October 2:

Time: _____   Blood Sugar: _____

Time: _____   Blood Sugar: _____

Time: _____   Blood Sugar: _____

Time: _____   Blood Sugar: _____

Wednesday, October 3:

Time: _____   Blood Sugar: _____

Time: _____   Blood Sugar: _____

Time: _____   Blood Sugar: _____

Time: _____   Blood Sugar: _____

Thursday, October 4:

Time: _____   Blood Sugar: _____

Time: _____   Blood Sugar: _____

Time: _____   Blood Sugar: _____

Time: _____   Blood Sugar: _____

Friday, October 5:

Time: _____   Blood Sugar: _____

Time: _____   Blood Sugar: _____

Time: _____   Blood Sugar: _____

Time: _____   Blood Sugar: _____

Saturday, October 6:

Time: _____   Blood Sugar: _____

Time: _____   Blood Sugar: _____

Time: _____   Blood Sugar: _____

Time: _____   Blood Sugar: _____

Sunday, October 7:

Time: _____   Blood Sugar: _____

Time: _____   Blood Sugar: _____

Time: _____   Blood Sugar: _____

Time: _____   Blood Sugar: _____

Monday, October 8:

Time: _____   Blood Sugar: _____

Time: _____   Blood Sugar: _____

Time: _____   Blood Sugar: _____

Time: _____   Blood Sugar: _____

Tuesday, October 9:

Time: _____   Blood Sugar: _____

Time: _____   Blood Sugar: _____

Time: _____   Blood Sugar: _____

Time: _____   Blood Sugar: _____

Wednesday, October 10:

Time: _____   Blood Sugar: _____

Time: _____   Blood Sugar: _____

Time: _____   Blood Sugar: _____

Time: _____   Blood Sugar: _____

Thursday, October 11:

Time: _____   Blood Sugar: _____

Time: _____   Blood Sugar: _____

Time: _____   Blood Sugar: _____

Time: _____   Blood Sugar: _____

Friday, October 12:

Time: _____   Blood Sugar: _____

Time: _____   Blood Sugar: _____

Time: _____   Blood Sugar: _____

Time: _____   Blood Sugar: _____

Saturday, October 13:

Time: _____   Blood Sugar: _____

Time: _____   Blood Sugar: _____

Time: _____   Blood Sugar: _____

Time: _____   Blood Sugar: _____

Sunday, October 14:

Time: _____   Blood Sugar: _____

Time: _____   Blood Sugar: _____

Time: _____   Blood Sugar: _____

Time: _____   Blood Sugar: _____

Monday, October 15:

Time: _____   Blood Sugar: _____

Time: _____   Blood Sugar: _____

Time: _____   Blood Sugar: _____

Time: _____   Blood Sugar: _____

Tuesday, October 16:

Time: _____   Blood Sugar: _____

Time: _____   Blood Sugar: _____

Time: _____   Blood Sugar: _____

Time: _____   Blood Sugar: _____

Wednesday, October 17:

Time: _____   Blood Sugar: _____

Time: _____   Blood Sugar: _____

Time: _____   Blood Sugar: _____

Time: _____   Blood Sugar: _____

Thursday, October 18:

Time: _____   Blood Sugar: _____

Time: _____   Blood Sugar: _____

Time: _____   Blood Sugar: _____

Time: _____   Blood Sugar: _____

Friday, October 19:

Time: _____   Blood Sugar: _____

Time: _____   Blood Sugar: _____

Time: _____   Blood Sugar: _____

Time: _____   Blood Sugar: _____

Saturday, October 20:

Time: _____   Blood Sugar: _____

Time: _____   Blood Sugar: _____

Time: _____   Blood Sugar: _____

Time: _____   Blood Sugar: _____

Sunday, October 21:

Time: _____   Blood Sugar: _____

Time: _____   Blood Sugar: _____

Time: _____   Blood Sugar: _____

Time: _____   Blood Sugar: _____

Monday, October 22:

Time: _____   Blood Sugar: _____

Time: _____   Blood Sugar: _____

Time: _____   Blood Sugar: _____

Time: _____   Blood Sugar: _____

Tuesday, October 23:

Time: _____   Blood Sugar: _____

Time: _____   Blood Sugar: _____

Time: _____   Blood Sugar: _____

Time: _____   Blood Sugar: _____

Wednesday, October 24:

Time: _____   Blood Sugar: _____

Time: _____   Blood Sugar: _____

Time: _____   Blood Sugar: _____

Time: _____   Blood Sugar: _____

Thursday, October 25:

Time: _____   Blood Sugar: _____

Time: _____   Blood Sugar: _____

Time: _____   Blood Sugar: _____

Time: _____   Blood Sugar: _____

Friday, October 26:

Time: _____   Blood Sugar: _____

Time: _____   Blood Sugar: _____

Time: _____   Blood Sugar: _____

Time: _____   Blood Sugar: _____

Saturday, October 27:

Time: _____ Blood Sugar: _____

Time: _____ Blood Sugar: _____

Time: _____ Blood Sugar: _____

Time: _____ Blood Sugar: _____

Sunday, October 28:

Time: _____ Blood Sugar: _____

Time: _____ Blood Sugar: _____

Time: _____ Blood Sugar: _____

Time: _____ Blood Sugar: _____

HOME BLOOD SUGAR
MONITORING RECORDS

November

Goals:

Morning (fasting) approximately = 100

Bedtime approximately = 140

After meals (2 hours) approximately = 140

Monday, October 29:

Time: _____   Blood Sugar: _____

Time: _____   Blood Sugar: _____

Time: _____   Blood Sugar: _____

Time: _____   Blood Sugar: _____

Tuesday, October 30:

Time: _____   Blood Sugar: _____

Time: _____   Blood Sugar: _____

Time: _____   Blood Sugar: _____

Time: _____   Blood Sugar: _____

Wednesday, October 31:

Time: _____   Blood Sugar: _____

Time: _____   Blood Sugar: _____

Time: _____   Blood Sugar: _____

Time: _____   Blood Sugar: _____

Thursday, November 1:

Time: _____   Blood Sugar: _____

Time: _____   Blood Sugar: _____

Time: _____   Blood Sugar: _____

Time: _____   Blood Sugar: _____

Friday, November 2:

Time: _____   Blood Sugar: _____

Time: _____   Blood Sugar: _____

Time: _____   Blood Sugar: _____

Time: _____   Blood Sugar: _____

Saturday, November 3:

Time: _____   Blood Sugar: _____

Time: _____   Blood Sugar: _____

Time: _____   Blood Sugar: _____

Time: _____   Blood Sugar: _____

Sunday, November 4:

Time: _____   Blood Sugar: _____

Time: _____   Blood Sugar: _____

Time: _____   Blood Sugar: _____

Time: _____   Blood Sugar: _____

Monday, November 5:

Time: _____   Blood Sugar: _____

Time: _____   Blood Sugar: _____

Time: _____   Blood Sugar: _____

Time: _____   Blood Sugar: _____

Tuesday, November 6:

Time: _____   Blood Sugar: _____

Time: _____   Blood Sugar: _____

Time: _____   Blood Sugar: _____

Time: _____   Blood Sugar: _____

Wednesday, November 7:

Time: _____   Blood Sugar: _____

Time: _____   Blood Sugar: _____

Time: _____   Blood Sugar: _____

Time: _____   Blood Sugar: _____

Thursday, November 8:

Time: _____   Blood Sugar: _____

Time: _____   Blood Sugar: _____

Time: _____   Blood Sugar: _____

Time: _____   Blood Sugar: _____

Friday, November 9:

Time: _____   Blood Sugar: _____

Time: _____   Blood Sugar: _____

Time: _____   Blood Sugar: _____

Time: _____   Blood Sugar: _____

Saturday, November 10:

Time: _____   Blood Sugar: _____

Time: _____   Blood Sugar: _____

Time: _____   Blood Sugar: _____

Time: _____   Blood Sugar: _____

Sunday, November 11:

Time: _____   Blood Sugar: _____

Time: _____   Blood Sugar: _____

Time: _____   Blood Sugar: _____

Time: _____   Blood Sugar: _____

Monday, November 12:

Time: _____   Blood Sugar: _____

Time: _____   Blood Sugar: _____

Time: _____   Blood Sugar: _____

Time: _____   Blood Sugar: _____

Tuesday, November 13:

Time: _____   Blood Sugar: _____

Time: _____   Blood Sugar: _____

Time: _____   Blood Sugar: _____

Time: _____   Blood Sugar: _____

Wednesday, November 14:

Time: _____   Blood Sugar: _____

Time: _____   Blood Sugar: _____

Time: _____   Blood Sugar: _____

Time: _____   Blood Sugar: _____

Thursday, November 15:

Time: _____   Blood Sugar: _____

Time: _____   Blood Sugar: _____

Time: _____   Blood Sugar: _____

Time: _____   Blood Sugar: _____

Friday, November 16:

Time: _____   Blood Sugar: _____

Time: _____   Blood Sugar: _____

Time: _____   Blood Sugar: _____

Time: _____   Blood Sugar: _____

Saturday, November 17:

Time: _____   Blood Sugar: _____

Time: _____   Blood Sugar: _____

Time: _____   Blood Sugar: _____

Time: _____   Blood Sugar: _____

Sunday, November 18:

Time: _____   Blood Sugar: _____

Time: _____   Blood Sugar: _____

Time: _____   Blood Sugar: _____

Time: _____   Blood Sugar: _____

Monday, November 19:

Time: _____   Blood Sugar: _____

Time: _____   Blood Sugar: _____

Time: _____   Blood Sugar: _____

Time: _____   Blood Sugar: _____

Tuesday, November 20:

Time: _____   Blood Sugar: _____

Time: _____   Blood Sugar: _____

Time: _____   Blood Sugar: _____

Time: _____   Blood Sugar: _____

Wednesday, November 21:

Time: _____   Blood Sugar: _____

Time: _____   Blood Sugar: _____

Time: _____   Blood Sugar: _____

Time: _____   Blood Sugar: _____

Thursday, November 22:

Time: _____   Blood Sugar: _____

Time: _____   Blood Sugar: _____

Time: _____   Blood Sugar: _____

Time: _____   Blood Sugar: _____

Friday, November 23:

Time: _____   Blood Sugar: _____

Time: _____   Blood Sugar: _____

Time: _____   Blood Sugar: _____

Time: _____   Blood Sugar: _____

Saturday, November 24:

Time: _____   Blood Sugar: _____

Time: _____   Blood Sugar: _____

Time: _____   Blood Sugar: _____

Time: _____   Blood Sugar: _____

Sunday, November 25:

Time: _____   Blood Sugar: _____

Time: _____   Blood Sugar: _____

Time: _____   Blood Sugar: _____

Time: _____   Blood Sugar: _____

Monday, November 26:

Time: _____ Blood Sugar: _____

Time: _____ Blood Sugar: _____

Time: _____ Blood Sugar: _____

Time: _____ Blood Sugar: _____

Tuesday, November 27:

Time: _____ Blood Sugar: _____

Time: _____ Blood Sugar: _____

Time: _____ Blood Sugar: _____

Time: _____ Blood Sugar: _____

Wednesday, November 28:

Time: _____ Blood Sugar: _____

Time: _____ Blood Sugar: _____

Time: _____ Blood Sugar: _____

Time: _____ Blood Sugar: _____

Thursday, November 29:

Time: _____ Blood Sugar: _____

Time: _____ Blood Sugar: _____

Time: _____ Blood Sugar: _____

Time: _____ Blood Sugar: _____

Friday, November 30:

Time: _____ Blood Sugar: _____

Time: _____ Blood Sugar: _____

Time: _____ Blood Sugar: _____

Time: _____ Blood Sugar: _____

Saturday, December 1:

Time: _____ Blood Sugar: _____

Time: _____ Blood Sugar: _____

Time: _____ Blood Sugar: _____

Time: _____ Blood Sugar: _____

Sunday, December 2:

Time: _____ Blood Sugar: _____

Time: _____ Blood Sugar: _____

Time: _____ Blood Sugar: _____

Time: _____ Blood Sugar: _____

HOME BLOOD SUGAR MONITORING RECORDS

December

Goals: Morning (fasting) approximately = 100

Bedtime approximately = 140

After meals (2 hours) approximately = 140

Monday, December 3:

Time: _____   Blood Sugar: _____

Time: _____   Blood Sugar: _____

Time: _____   Blood Sugar: _____

Time: _____   Blood Sugar: _____

Tuesday, December 4:

Time: _____   Blood Sugar: _____

Time: _____   Blood Sugar: _____

Time: _____   Blood Sugar: _____

Time: _____   Blood Sugar: _____

Wednesday, December 5:

Time: _____   Blood Sugar: _____

Time: _____   Blood Sugar: _____

Time: _____   Blood Sugar: _____

Time: _____   Blood Sugar: _____

Thursday, December 6:

Time: _____   Blood Sugar: _____

Time: _____   Blood Sugar: _____

Time: _____   Blood Sugar: _____

Time: _____   Blood Sugar: _____

Friday, December 7:

Time: _____   Blood Sugar: _____

Time: _____   Blood Sugar: _____

Time: _____   Blood Sugar: _____

Time: _____   Blood Sugar: _____

Saturday, December 8:

Time: _____   Blood Sugar: _____

Time: _____   Blood Sugar: _____

Time: _____   Blood Sugar: _____

Time: _____   Blood Sugar: _____

Sunday, December 9:

Time: _____   Blood Sugar: _____

Time: _____   Blood Sugar: _____

Time: _____   Blood Sugar: _____

Time: _____   Blood Sugar: _____

Monday, December 10:

Time: _____ Blood Sugar: _____

Time: _____ Blood Sugar: _____

Time: _____ Blood Sugar: _____

Time: _____ Blood Sugar: _____

Tuesday, December 11:

Time: _____ Blood Sugar: _____

Time: _____ Blood Sugar: _____

Time: _____ Blood Sugar: _____

Time: _____ Blood Sugar: _____

Wednesday, December 12:

Time: _____ Blood Sugar: _____

Time: _____ Blood Sugar: _____

Time: _____ Blood Sugar: _____

Time: _____ Blood Sugar: _____

Thursday, December 13:

Time: _____ Blood Sugar: _____

Time: _____ Blood Sugar: _____

Time: _____ Blood Sugar: _____

Time: _____ Blood Sugar: _____

Friday, December 14:

Time: _____ Blood Sugar: _____

Time: _____ Blood Sugar: _____

Time: _____ Blood Sugar: _____

Time: _____ Blood Sugar: _____

Saturday, December 15:

Time: _____   Blood Sugar: _____

Time: _____   Blood Sugar: _____

Time: _____   Blood Sugar: _____

Time: _____   Blood Sugar: _____

Sunday, December 16:

Time: _____   Blood Sugar: _____

Time: _____   Blood Sugar: _____

Time: _____   Blood Sugar: _____

Time: _____   Blood Sugar: _____

Monday, December 17:

Time: _____   Blood Sugar: _____

Time: _____   Blood Sugar: _____

Time: _____   Blood Sugar: _____

Time: _____   Blood Sugar: _____

Tuesday, December 18:

Time: _____   Blood Sugar: _____

Time: _____   Blood Sugar: _____

Time: _____   Blood Sugar: _____

Time: _____   Blood Sugar: _____

Wednesday, December 19:

Time: _____   Blood Sugar: _____

Time: _____   Blood Sugar: _____

Time: _____   Blood Sugar: _____

Time: _____   Blood Sugar: _____

Thursday, December 20:

Time: _____   Blood Sugar: _____

Time: _____   Blood Sugar: _____

Time: _____   Blood Sugar: _____

Time: _____   Blood Sugar: _____

Friday, December 21:

Time: _____   Blood Sugar: _____

Time: _____   Blood Sugar: _____

Time: _____   Blood Sugar: _____

Time: _____   Blood Sugar: _____

Saturday, December 22:

Time: _____   Blood Sugar: _____

Time: _____   Blood Sugar: _____

Time: _____   Blood Sugar: _____

Time: _____   Blood Sugar: _____

Sunday, December 23:

Time: _____   Blood Sugar: _____

Time: _____   Blood Sugar: _____

Time: _____   Blood Sugar: _____

Time: _____   Blood Sugar: _____

Monday, December 24:

Time: _____ Blood Sugar: _____

Time: _____ Blood Sugar: _____

Time: _____ Blood Sugar: _____

Time: _____ Blood Sugar: _____

Tuesday, December 25:

Time: _____ Blood Sugar: _____

Time: _____ Blood Sugar: _____

Time: _____ Blood Sugar: _____

Time: _____ Blood Sugar: _____

Wednesday, December 26:

Time: _____ Blood Sugar: _____

Time: _____ Blood Sugar: _____

Time: _____ Blood Sugar: _____

Time: _____ Blood Sugar: _____

Thursday, December 27:

Time: _____ Blood Sugar: _____

Time: _____ Blood Sugar: _____

Time: _____ Blood Sugar: _____

Time: _____ Blood Sugar: _____

Friday, December 28:

Time: _____ Blood Sugar: _____

Time: _____ Blood Sugar: _____

Time: _____ Blood Sugar: _____

Time: _____ Blood Sugar: _____

Saturday, December 29:

Time: _____   Blood Sugar: _____

Time: _____   Blood Sugar: _____

Time: _____   Blood Sugar: _____

Time: _____   Blood Sugar: _____

Sunday, December 30:

Time: _____   Blood Sugar: _____

Time: _____   Blood Sugar: _____

Time: _____   Blood Sugar: _____

Time: _____   Blood Sugar: _____

Monday, December 31:

Time: _____   Blood Sugar: _____

Time: _____   Blood Sugar: _____

Time: _____   Blood Sugar: _____

Time: _____   Blood Sugar: _____

Tuesday, January 2, 2002:

Time: _____   Blood Sugar: _____

Time: _____   Blood Sugar: _____

Time: _____   Blood Sugar: _____

Time: _____   Blood Sugar: _____

Wednesday, January 2, 2002:

Time: _____   Blood Sugar: _____

Time: _____   Blood Sugar: _____

Time: _____   Blood Sugar: _____

Time: _____   Blood Sugar: _____

Thursday, January 3, 2002:

Time: _____   Blood Sugar: _____

Time: _____   Blood Sugar: _____

Time: _____   Blood Sugar: _____

Time: _____   Blood Sugar: _____

Friday, January 4, 2002:

Time: _____   Blood Sugar: _____

Time: _____   Blood Sugar: _____

Time: _____   Blood Sugar: _____

Time: _____   Blood Sugar: _____

Saturday, January 5, 2002:

Time: _____ Blood Sugar: _____

Time: _____ Blood Sugar: _____

Time: _____ Blood Sugar: _____

Time: _____ Blood Sugar: _____

Sunday, January 6, 2002:

Time: _____ Blood Sugar: _____

Time: _____ Blood Sugar: _____

Time: _____ Blood Sugar: _____

Time: _____ Blood Sugar: _____

WEIGHTS

▶ Checks for risk of worsening diabetes.

▶ Recording your weights monthly should be adequate.

▶ Weight management is important, especially in Type 2 diabetes. Obese Type 2 diabetics can significantly improve their blood sugar control and even cure their diabetes with weight reduction. Conversely, weight gain can contribute to uncontrolled diabetes and subsequent complications.

▶ Calculate your body mass index (BMI) from the following formula:
BMI = weight _____ Kg ÷ (height _____ meters)^2
Normal is BMI ≤ 25.
Overweight is BMI between 25 and 30.
Obese is BMI ≥ 30.

▶ Conversion from English units is easy.
Weight _____ lb. ÷ 2.2 = _____ Kg.
Height _____ in. x 2.54 ÷ 100 = _____ meters.

WEIGHTS

January:

_____ lb.

_____ Kg.

_____ BMI

February:

_____ lb.

_____ Kg.

_____ BMI

March:

_____ lb.

_____ Kg.

_____ BMI

April:

_____ lb.

_____ Kg.

_____ BMI

May:

_____ lb.

_____ Kg.

_____ BMI

June:

_____ lb.

_____ Kg.

_____ BMI

July:

_____ lb.

_____ Kg.

_____ BMI

August:

_____ lb.

_____ Kg.

_____ BMI

September:

_____ lb.

_____ Kg.

_____ BMI

October:

_____ lb.

_____ Kg.

_____ BMI

November:

_____ lb.

_____ Kg.

_____ BMI

December:

_____ lb.

_____ Kg.

_____ BMI

BLOOD PRESSURE

▶ Checks risk for heart disease, stroke and kidney disease.
▶ Record your blood pressures as measured by a health care professional monthly should be adequate. Your physician may monitor your blood pressure more frequently until it is under control. You may use an average if your health care provider measures several readings during one visit.
▶ Current recommendations:
Systolic Blood Pressure $\leq$ **135** (top number).
Diastolic Blood Pressure $\leq$ **85** (bottom number).

BLOOD PRESSURE

January:

_____

mm Hg Systolic

_____

mm Hg Diastolic

February:

_____

mm Hg Systolic

_____

mm Hg Diastolic

March:

_____

mm Hg Systolic

_____

mm Hg Diastolic

April:

_____

mm Hg Systolic

_____

mm Hg Diastolic

May:

_____

mm Hg Systolic

_____

mm Hg Diastolic

June:

_____

mm Hg Systolic

_____

mm Hg Diastolic

July:

_____

mm Hg Systolic

_____

mm Hg Diastolic

August:

_____

mm Hg Systolic

_____

mm Hg Diastolic

September:

_____

mm Hg Systolic

_____

mm Hg Diastolic

October:

_____

mm Hg Systolic

_____

mm Hg Diastolic
November:

_____

mm Hg Systolic

_____

mm Hg Diastolic
December:

_____

mm Hg Systolic

_____

mm Hg Diastolic

HEMOGLOBIN A₁C
(GLYCOSYLATED HEMOGLOBIN)

▶ Measures average blood sugar control over the preceding 2 or 3 months.

▶ Record values in the corresponding month in which they were tested.

▶ Measurement is recommended twice yearly if sugar control is stable and quarterly if treatment goals aren't met or if therapy is changed.

▶ **As a general rule, therapeutic blood sugar control is indicated by a result of ≤ 7%. Change in therapy is indicated at values ≥ 8%.**

▶ Note: There is a lack of standardization between assays, so your doctor may make recommendations idiosyncratic to the assay used.

HEMOGLOBIN A$_1$C
(GLYCOSYLATED HEMOGLOBIN)

January: ...._____ %

February: ...._____ %

March: ...._____ %

April:..............._____ %

May: ...._____ %

June: ...._____ %

July: ...._____ %

August: ...._____ %

September:......_____ %

October: ...._____ %

November: ......_____ %

December: ......_____ %

LIPIDS

▶ Checks risk for heart disease and stroke.

▶ Record values in the corresponding month in which they were tested.

▶ Generally, adult diabetic patients should have their lipids checked yearly. Lipids that should be measured include LDL-cholesterol (bad cholesterol), HDL-cholesterol (good cholesterol) and triglycerides.

▶ If the resultant values fall into the low risk category (LDL-C < 100 mg/dL, HDL-C > 45 mg/dL for men and > 55 mg/dL for women, triglycerides <200) screening can be performed every 2 years.

▶ Testing may be indicated more often when being pharmacologically treated for high risk lipid levels, especially in the initiation stages.

▶ Therapeutic goals include
LDL-cholesterol < 100 mg/dL
HDL-cholesterol > 45 mg/dL for men and >55 mg/dL for women
Triglycerides < 400 mg/dL (< 200 may be beneficial)

▶ If treated pharmacologically other tests may be indicated, most commonly the transaminases ALT (alanine aminotransferase) and AST (aspartame aminotransferase) to monitor liver function and CK (creatine kinase) to monitor skeletal muscle biochemistry. Space is included for these test results.

LIPIDS

January:

LDL-C ._____ mg/dl   ALT....._____ IU/dl

HDL-C _____ mg/dl   AST ...._____ IU/dl

Trig......._____ mg/dl   CK......_____ IU/dl

February:

LDL-C ._____ mg/dl   ALT....._____ IU/dl

HDL-C _____ mg/dl   AST ...._____ IU/dl

Trig......._____ mg/dl   CK......_____ IU/dl

March:

LDL-C ._____ mg/dl   ALT....._____ IU/dl

HDL-C _____ mg/dl   AST ...._____ IU/dl

Trig......._____ mg/dl   CK......_____ IU/dl

April:

LDL-C ._____ mg/dl   ALT....._____ IU/dl

HDL-C _____ mg/dl   AST ...._____ IU/dl

Trig......._____ mg/dl   CK......_____ IU/dl

May:

LDL-C _____ mg/dl   ALT _____ IU/dl

HDL-C _____ mg/dl   AST _____ IU/dl

Trig. _____ mg/dl   CK _____ IU/dl

June:

LDL-C	_____ mg/dl		ALT	_____ IU/dl	
HDL-C	_____ mg/dl		AST	_____ IU/dl	
Trig.	_____ mg/dl		CK	_____ IU/dl	

July:

LDL-C ._____ mg/dl   ALT....._____ IU/dl

HDL-C _____ mg/dl   AST ...._____ IU/dl

Trig......._____ mg/dl   CK......_____ IU/dl

August:

LDL-C ._____ mg/dl   ALT....._____ IU/dl

HDL-C _____ mg/dl   AST ...._____ IU/dl

Trig......._____ mg/dl   CK......_____ IU/dl

September:

LDL-C ._____ mg/dl   ALT....._____ IU/dl

HDL-C _____ mg/dl   AST ...._____ IU/dl

Trig......._____ mg/dl   CK......_____ IU/dl

October:

LDL-C ._____ mg/dl   ALT....._____ IU/dl

HDL-C _____ mg/dl   AST ...._____ IU/dl

Trig......._____ mg/dl   CK......_____ IU/dl

November:

LDL-C	_____ mg/dl		ALT	_____ IU/dl	
HDL-C	_____ mg/dl		AST	_____ IU/dl	
Trig.	_____ mg/dl		CK	_____ IU/dl	

December:

LDL-C	_____ mg/dl	ALT	_____ IU/dl
HDL-C	_____ mg/dl	AST	_____ IU/dl
Trig.	_____ mg/dl	CK	_____ IU/dl

Urinary Microalbumin

▶ Checks kidney (renal function)
▶ Record values in the corresponding month in which they were tested.
▶ Urinalysis should be performed yearly. If no protein is detected then a follow up test should be performed looking for small amounts of albumin, called microalbumin. The test can be performed in any of three ways.

1. Random first morning urine sample is the most common and convenient method used. The creatinine in the urine is also measured and the result is reported as a ratio. If a first morning specimen is not possible, urine samples should be obtained at the same time of day for meaningful comparisons.
   Normal value is < 30 μg/mg.
2. Twenty four hour collection. Urine is collected for 24 hours and analyzed for the total albumin. Your physician may also order a creatinine clearance test simultaneously to check your kidney function.
   Normal value is <30 mg/24 hr.
3. Timed collection over 4 or 8 hours.
   Normal value is <20 μg/min.

▶ Because of normal variability, 2 of 3 specimens over a 3 to 6 month period should be abnormal before this test is considered positive. Exercise, infection, fever, congestive heart failure, severe hyperglycemia and severe hypertension can cause false positives.

▶ If you have been diagnosed with gross protein in your urine (proteinuria) no microalbumin testing is indicated. Just check the space provided for gross proteinuria.

URINARY MICROALBUMIN

Check here if gross proteinuria _____

January:

_____ μg/mg

_____ mg/hr

_____ μg/min

February:

_____ μg/mg

_____ mg/hr

_____ μg/min

March:

_____ μg/mg

_____ mg/hr

_____ μg/min

April:

_____ μg/mg

_____ mg/hr

_____ μg/min

May:

_____ μg/mg

_____ mg/hr

_____ μg/min

June:

_____ µg/mg

_____ mg/hr

_____ µg/min

July:

_____ µg/mg

_____ mg/hr

_____ µg/min

August:

_____ µg/mg

_____ mg/hr

_____ µg/min

September:

_____ µg/mg

_____ mg/hr

_____ µg/min

October:

_____ µg/mg

_____ mg/hr

_____ µg/min

November:

_____ µg/mg

_____ mg/hr

_____ µg/min

December:

_____ µg/mg

_____ mg/hr

_____ µg/min

KIDNEY (RENAL) FUNCTION

▶ Record values in the corresponding month in which they were tested.

▶ Another measurement of kidney function is blood urea nitrogen (BUN) and creatinine (CRT). Especially if you are taking a blood pressure medication called ACE inhibitors (angiotensin converting enzyme inhibitors) you should have your BUN, CRT and K (potassium) checked 2-3 weeks after initiation of the medication and 2-3 weeks after any dose change, then periodically.

KIDNEY (RENAL) FUNCTION

January:

BUN.._____ mg/dl

CRT .._____ mg/dl

K ...._____ meq/dl

February:

BUN.._____ mg/dl

CRT .._____ mg/dl

K ...._____ meq/dl

March:

BUN.._____ mg/dl

CRT .._____ mg/dl

K ...._____ meq/dl

April:

BUN.._____ mg/dl

CRT .._____ mg/dl

K ...._____ meq/dl

May:

BUN.._____ mg/dl

CRT .._____ mg/dl

K ...._____ meq/dl

June:

BUN.._____ mg/dl

CRT .._____ mg/dl

K ...._____ meq/dl

July:

BUN.._____ mg/dl

CRT .._____ mg/dl

K ...._____ meq/dl

August:

BUN.._____ mg/dl

CRT .._____ mg/dl

K ...._____ meq/dl

September:

BUN.._____ mg/dl

CRT .._____ mg/dl

K ...._____ meq/dl

October:

BUN.._____ mg/dl

CRT .._____ mg/dl

K ...._____ meq/dl

November:

BUN.._____ mg/dl

CRT .._____ mg/dl

K ...._____ meq/dl

December:

BUN.._____ mg/dl

CRT .._____ mg/dl

K ...._____ meq/dl

EXAMINATIONS

▶ Record the physician number in the month examined.
▶ Enter the names of your physicians below the table and the dates of last year's most recent examination with them.
▶ General diabetic examinations:
Twice yearly if controlled.
Quarterly if not meeting therapeutic goals. More often if prescribed.
▶ Foot examinations should be performed at every doctor visit. **It is best just to get into the habit of taking your shoes and socks off every time you see your doctor!** Some recommend at least a yearly examination by a foot specialist such as a podiatrist, orthopedic surgeon or vascular surgeon.
▶ **Diabetic eye examinations should be performed yearly by an ophthalmologist**; more often if prescribed. Diabetes is still the most common cause of blindness world wide.

EXAMINATIONS

January:

_____ Diabetic

_____ Foot

_____ Opthalmologic

February:

_____ Diabetic

_____ Foot

_____ Opthalmologic

March:

_____ Diabetic

_____ Foot

_____ Opthalmologic

April:

_____ Diabetic

_____ Foot

_____ Opthalmologic

May:

_____ Diabetic

_____ Foot

_____ Opthalmologic

June:

_____ Diabetic

_____ Foot

_____ Opthalmologic

July:

_____ Diabetic

_____ Foot

_____ Opthalmologic

August:

_____ Diabetic

_____ Foot

_____ Opthalmologic

September:

_____ Diabetic

_____ Foot

_____ Opthalmologic

October:

_____ Diabetic

_____ Foot

_____ Opthalmologic

November:

_____ Diabetic

_____ Foot

_____ Opthalmologic

December:

_____ Diabetic

_____ Foot

_____ Opthalmologic

1. Primary Cary Doctor_____

2. Diabetic specialist (if different) _____

3. Ophthalmologist_____

4. Foot specialist   _____

REFERENCES

1. American Diabetic Association. *www.diabetes.org.* December 2000 review of Position statements, Consensus statements and Technical reviews.
2. ABCNEWS.com. Fending off the Flu, New Pill Works Like Vaccine, 20 November 2000.
3. American Family Physician. Alternative Therapies: Part I. Depression, Diabetes, Obesity. 1 September 2000.
4. American Family Physician. Diagnosis and Classification of Diabetes Mellitus New Criteria. 15 October 1998
5. American Family Physician. New Oral Therapies for Type 2 Diabetes. 1 November 1997.
6. American Family Physician. New Treatments for Diabetes. 15 May 1999.
7. American Family Physician. Oral Pharmacological of Type 2 Diabetes. 1 December 1999.
8. American Family Physician. Use of ACE Inhibitors in Patients with Type 2 Diabetes. 1 May 2000.

ABOUT THE AUTHOR

L. D. Sutton, M.D., Ph.D.

Dr. Sutton is a physician-scientist with 58 scientific publications and presentations to his credit. He received his Medical Degree from the University of Iowa College of Medicine and his Doctoral degree from the University of Iowa College of Liberal Arts' Department of Chemistry. He completed specialty training in Clinical Pathology at the University of Iowa Hospitals and Clinics and in Family Practice at Broadlawns Medical Center in Des Moines, Iowa. His practice experience includes faculty positions in pathology at both the University of Arkansas for Medical Sciences and the University of Iowa Hospitals and Clinics, Director of Clinical Microbiology at the McClellan Memorial Veteran's Administration Hospital in Little Rock, Arkansas and a successful private practice in Family and Emergency Medicine. After serving as Senior Research Scientist for Bio-Research Products, Inc., he co-founded Joel Health Industries, Inc. where he currently works as President.

www.ingramcontent.com/pod-product-compliance
Lightning Source LLC
Chambersburg PA
CBHW020918290526
45784CB00002BA/611